Gaps Diet

Recipes For Alleviating Chronic Inflammation, Repairing
The Gut Wall, And Regaining Energy

(Gaps Diet Cookbook For Beginners)

Delbert Osborne

TABLE OF CONTENT

Chapter 1: What Is The Gaps Diet?

The GAPS Diet excludes cereals, pasteurized dairy, starchy vegetables, and refined carbohydrates, among other foods. According to the GAPS diet theory, avoiding specific foods will improve digestive health, which can ultimately benefit individuals with dyslexia, autism, and Attention-Deficit/Hyperactivity Disorder (ADHD).

The GAPS diet is not a weight reduction plan; it is a restrictive diet designed to treat mental health conditions such as dyslexia, attention deficit hyperactivity disorder (ADHD), and autism spectrum disorder (ASD).Many individuals with autism commonly experience diarrhea, constipation, and abdominal distention. The acronym for "gut and psychology syndrome" is "GAPS." The GAPS diet was created by Natasha Campbell-McBride, MD, a physician and author with additional postgraduate degrees in nutrition and neurology.

After her son was diagnosed with autism, she used her expertise to devise a probable nutrition-based treatment for him. The Specific Carbohydrate Diet (SCD), used to treat celiac disease, Crohn's disease, ulcerative colitis, and inflammatory bowel disease, is the basis for the GAPS diet, which prohibits all grains, sugar, and simple carbohydrates. In a similar manner, the GAPS diet uses fermented vegetables and prepared broths to treat intestinal permeability, also known as "leaky gut syndrome."

Chapter 2: Which conditions is the Gaps Diet designed to treat?

Some people also use the GAPS diet as an alternative treatment for a number of mental and behavioral disorders, such as disordered eating, childhood food intolerances and allergies, autism, ADHD, dyslexia, dyspraxia, epilepsy, depression, schizophrenia, bipolar disorder, and obsessive-compulsive disorder (OCD).

Chapter 3: The Gaps Diet And Autism

Autism develops in children with leaky gastrointestinal syndrome and inadequate nutrition. She claims that the GAPS diet can "cure" or mitigate symptoms of autism. As a consequence of ASD, a variety of symptoms impact a person's worldview and social interactions.According to scientists, ASD is caused by a combination of genetic and environmental factors. The consensus among experts is that ASD cannot be treated. However, it is feasible to treat health issues associated with ASD, such as gastrointestinal (GI) issues. Significantly more children with ASD exhibited gastrointestinal symptoms than children without ASD. Children with ASD were more likely to experience diarrhea, constipation, and abdominal distress, according to the authors.

BENEFIT OF FOLLOWING A GAPS DIET

There is no evidence that the GAPS diet can treat all of the conditions for which it is promoted. However, following this diet may enhance a person's gut health. It encourages the consumption of more natural lipids, fruits, and vegetables as opposed to processed foods. The health of the intestine and the entire body may benefit from these simple dietary modifications. To avoid nutrient deficiency, individuals following this diet should consume sufficient vitamins and minerals.

A healthy gut contributes to a robust immune system, heart health, mental health, improved mood, restful sleep, and efficient digestion.

Aid in the prevention of certain malignancies and autoimmune disorders.

STOP USING ARTIFICIAL SWEETENERS: Artificial sweeteners have the potential to cause intestinal bacteria imbalances and increase the risk of metabolic disorders.

Simply Prepared Mayonnaise

- 1/2 teaspoon of mustard, chili, or chipotle powder (optional)
- 2 tablespoon of apple cider vinegar
- 1/2 teaspoon of sea salt
- 2 fresh, pastured organic fresh egg
- 2 cup of avocado oil or olive oil
  2

Directions

1. Firstly, pour oil into a liquid measuring cup and put aside.

2. Next, place egg, vinegar and salt and in a twelve-ounces mason jar.

3. Place 2 beater in a hand mixer and beat on high speed.

4. Next, pour in the oil while still beating on high for few minutes.

5. Next, add chili powder or mustard, if desired.

6. You can store covered in the fridge for about 2 month.

- Recipe for Low Carb Hamburger Soup Simple cook 2 (twenty-eight ounces) can diced tomatoes
- 4 carrots, sliced
- Eight cups of b2 broth
- 2 to half cup of green beans and/or asparagus, cut into 2 to half-inch pieces
- 2 green bell pepper, chopped
- Four cloves of garlic
- 4 cups of spinach packed
- Pepper, to taste
- Salt, to taste
- 4 pounds of ground beef

- 4 tablespoons of healthy fat such as ghee, lard or butter
- 2 teaspoon celery seed (optional)
- 2 onion, diced

Directions

1. In a soup saucepan with a thick bottom, melt your preferred fat over medium to high heat.

2. Then, add the onions and sauté them until they become translucent.

3. Add minced beef and simple cook it for approximately 10 to 15 minutes while breaking it up.

4. Next, stir in the diced tomatoes, celery seed, carrots, and broth, and bring to a simmer.

5. Simple reduce the heat to medium and simple cook for ten minutes, or until the carrots are tender.

6. Next, add the asparagus or green beans, followed by the bell pepper, and simmer for an additional five minutes.

1. simple cook simple cook simple cook simple cook Next, put off the heat, add garlic, spinach and then adjust salt and pepper, if necessary.

2. Stir to combine well.

3. Serve straightaway

4. Leftovers can be stored in refrigerator for about seven days.

Instant Pot Gaps Diet Introduction Soup

Ingredients

6 tablespoons lard or tallow

10 to 7 cloves garlic fresh, peeled

sea salt to taste

ground black pepper to taste

garnish cooked b2 marrow, sauerkraut juice, and/or sour cream 8   cups butternut squash peeled and cubed

2   pound cauliflower florets fresh or frozen

3 cups onion diced

2 cup orange pepper or yellow, diced

2 cup bone broth

Instructions

1. Add the squash, cauliflower florets, onion, pepper, broth, and fat to the stainless steel insert of your pressure cooker.

2. Place the lid on, checking the seal and making sure the vent is sealed.

3. If using an electric cooker, set to high pressure for 10 to 15 minutes.

4. If using a stove-top cooker, bring to high pressure and maintain for 10 to 15 minutes.

5. When cycle is complete, turn off or easily remove from heat.

6. Quick release pressure.

7. Add the garlic cloves to the pot.

8. Using an immersion blender, blend the soup to your desired consistency.

9. Season with salt and pepper to taste.

Dijon Tofu Ciabatta

Ingredients

- 60 grams Dijon mustard

- 2 tablespoon soy sauce

- 100 ml Extra virgin olive oil

- 2 teaspoon smoky paprika

- Salt and pepper to taste

- 8 crusty white ciabatta rolls • 2 zip

lock bag to marinate the tofu in

- 800 grams tofu cut into 2 00 grams

slabs

- 1 ripe avocado peeled and mashed

- 100 grams baby spinach leaves

- 8 slices tasty cheddar

- 60 ml lemon juice

- 60 grams whole egg mayonnaise

Directions

1. Season the tofu with salt and pepper – rub it in

2. Add 100 ml of olive oil, smokey paprika, fresh lemon juice, and soy sauce into a ziplocked bag, add the tofu and coat with the marinade, leave in the fridge of 2-2 1 hours.

3. Warm the BBQ to medium heat.

4. Add 60 grams of Dijon mustard to whole fresh egg mayonnaise and blend thoroughly.

5. Just take the tofu out of the fridge and out of the bag, grill each side of 5-10 minutes until golden.

6. Spread one side of each roll with Dijon/mayonnaise mix and the other side with mashed avocado.

7. Place a slice of cheese on the mayonnaise side and baby spinach leaves on the avocado side, press down slightly so they are a little embedded in the avocado.

8. Slice the tofu in thin strips and pile them evenly on the rocket side of each roll and close the roll.

9. Serve immediately.

Breakfast Bars With Coconut Flour, Blueberries, And Bananas

Simple cook Ingredients

• 8 bananas very ripe with spots

• 2 cup coconut flour

• 2 teaspoon baking soda

• 1 teaspoon sea salt

• 10-15 ounces of fresh or frozen
blueberries organic if possible

- 14 fresh eggs preferably pastured

- 8 tablespoons coconut oil

- 4 tablespoons honey

- 4 teaspoons vanilla

Instructions

1. Puree the bananas in a food processor or blender, then add the fresh eggs and continue to process until well mixed.

2. Add honey, oil, and vanilla. Blend well.

3. Add flour, baking soda and salt and blend until smooth.

4. Pour batter into a mixing bowl and add the blueberries, stirring well.

5. Grease a 10x15 pan and line it with parchment paper.

6. Pour batter into the pan and bake at 350 degrees Fahrenheit for 60 minutes.

7. Check the bars to see if the top is getting too brown at this point.

8. If it is, cover it with tin foil then continue to bake the bars for 20 more minutes.

Sweet Marinara Sauce From Ed Giobbi

Ingeredients

4 large cloves garlic, minced

8 cups fresh tomatoes, chopped; or

4 jars or cans (28 ounces each)

2 tablespoon chopped fresh basil

2 teaspoon dried oregano

Sea salt and freshly ground black pepper

6 tablespoons ghee, butter, or preferred fat, divided

2 medium onion, diced

4 medium carrots, chopped

Instructions

1. Heat 2 tablespoon of the ghee, butter, or preferred fat in a large saucepan over medium heat. Sauté the onion, carrots, and garlic until soft, about 20 minutes.

2. Add the tomatoes and easy simple cook for 30 minutes, until the sauce is bubbling.

3. Then simple reduce the heat to a simmer.

4. For a smooth sauce, zap with an immersion blender.

5. Throw in the herbs, season with salt and pepper, then easy simple cook for another 25 to 30 minutes.

6. Finally, add the remaining 4 tablespoons fat and stir until melted.

Red Bell Pepper Omelette

INGREDIENTS

- 1 cup cheese

- 1 tsp basil

- 2 cup red bell pepper
- **4 fresh eggs**

- 1 tsp salt

- 1 tsp black pepper

- 2 tablespoon olive oil

DIRECTIONS

1. In a bowl combine all ingredients together and mix well

2. In a skillet heat olive oil and pour the fresh egg mixture

3. Simple cook for 1-5 minutes per side

4. When ready easily remove omelette from the skillet and serve

Making Bone Broth in an Instant Pot

Ingredients

1 gallon water

2 tablespoon apple cider vinegar

Bones from a whole chicken

Vegetable Scraps

Instructions

1. Add the bones and any vegetable scraps to the instant pot.

2. Cover the bones with filtered water. I use the Berkey filter.

3. Add 2 tablespoon of apple cider vinegar.

4. Set it on the soup setting for 50 to 55 minutes.

5. When it is done, let it release pressure naturally.

6. Strain the bones off from the broth.

7. Store in an airtight container.

Flipped Fish And Chips

Ingredients

- 1 cup packed, chopped continental parsley

- 2 fresh lemon rind

- ground pepper

- 1400 grams white fish • 8 large, peeled red skinned potatoes

- olive oil spray

- 1 cup milk of your choice

- 1/2 cup plain white breadcrumbs

- 1/2 cup plain white flour

fresh lemon

Directions

1. Preheat fan forced oven to 250C

2. Line 4 large baking trays with baking paper

3. Put flour on a plate, milk in a wide bowl, and mix breadcrumbs parsley, lemon rind and pinch of ground pepper in a third wide bowl

4. Dip each piece of fish in flour, dust off excess coat thoroughly, then dip in milk and press into the breadcrumb mix until coated evenly

5. Place the piece of fish on the lined tray spray with olive oil on both sides

6. Repeat until all fish adequately coated – place them on a one of the lined oven trays

7. Place the chips in an oven bag and microwave for 5-10 minutes until tender

8. Just take them out and pat them dry with a paper cloth

9. Put them in a deep wide bowl

10. Spray them with oil and mix through salt and pepper to desired amount

11. Bake both fish and chips in the oven

12. Flip the fish and chips over once or twice to ensure they are both golden brown on both sides

13. Serve with favourite sauces and a green salad

Greens And Bacon Sunshine Frittata: Convenient And Delectable

Simple cook

Ingredients

- 1/2   cup coconut milk cream, or yogurt

- 1/2   teaspoon freshly ground black pepper

- 1/2   teaspoon turmeric

- 4 slices bacon cut into 1 inch slices

- 2 onion chopped

- 12 mushrooms sliced

- 8 cups loosely packed greens

- 24 eggs

Instructions

1. In a large cast iron skillet over medium heat, sautee
2. bacon for 5-10 minutes, or until it starts to release the
3. grease.
4. Add in mushrooms and onion and continue to
5. sautee until bacon is crisp and onions are translucent.
6. Dump in greens, and stir until wilted, about 5-10 more minutes.

7. Preheat oven to 350 * F

8. Gently mix fresh eggs with coconut milk, pepper and turmeric.

9. Pour over spinach mixture and put the whole pan in the oven.

10. Easily Easily remove from oven when center of the

11. fritatta is set and has puffed up a bit, about 35 to 40 minutes.

12. Top with cheese and return to the oven for 5-10

13. minutes, or until melted.

14. Slice into wedges and enjoy!

Breakfast Granola

INGREDIENTS

- 2 tablespoon honey

- 2 lb. rolled oats

- 4 tablespoons sesame seeds

- 1 lb. almonds

- 1 lb. berries

- 2 tsp vanilla extract

DIRECTIONS

1. Preheat the oven to 350 F
2. Spread the granola onto a baking sheet

3. Bake for 25 to 30 minutes, easily remove and mix everything

4. Bake for another 25 to 30 minutes or until slightly brown

5. When ready easily remove from the oven and serve

Keto Chili

Ingredients

6 cups strained tomatoes

2 Tbl apple cider vinegar

2 -6 Tbl chili powder

sea salt to taste

15-20 pounds ground beef preferably
grassfed

2 cup dried navy beans preferably
sprouted

Instructions

1. Place navy beans in a medium glass bowl and cover with filtered water.

2. Stir in a tablespoon of ACV and let sit overnight or up to 20 to 24 hours.

3. Drain navy beans, rinse thoroughly, and place in a large pot.

4. Cover with fresh water and then bring to a low boil on the stovetop.

5. Cover and turn down the heat. Simmer for one hour or until the navy beans are soft.

6. When the navy beans are soft, drain the water, rinse/drain with fresh water one more time, and set aside.

7. Saute ground beef until just cooked through in a large skillet.

8. Do NOT drain the fat. It is GOOD for you and very healing to the gut lining.

9. Add cooked navy beans and strained tomatoes.

10.   Stir on medium heat until hot.

11.   Mix in chili powder and sea salt to taste.

12.   Serve immediately.

13. Once cooled, refrigerate and enjoy as leftovers for up to four days.

Cauliflower Twist Soup

Ingredients:

- 4 cups boneless Organic Chicken, in bite-sized pieces
- 6 cups Cauliflower Florets, chopped roughly
- Natural unprocessed Salt, to taste
- Freshly Crushed Black Pepper, to taste

- 2 small Onion, chopped
- 6 Carrots, peeled and chopped
- 6 Garlic Cloves, minced
- 12 cups Homemade Chicken Broth

Instruction:

1. In a large soup pan, add the broth and chicken, and bring to boiling point on a high heat.

2. Reduce the heat, cover, and simmer for 15 to 20 minutes.

3. Add the onion, carrot, garlic and cauliflower, and bring to boiling point again.

4. Simple reduce the heat, cover, and simmer for a further 25 to 30 minutes.

5. Season with salt and black pepper before serving.

Tomato Chi Soup

Ingredients:

- 4 Zucchinis, peeled, seeded and chopped
- Natural unprocessed Salt, to taste
- Freshly Crushed Black Pepper, to taste
- 2 small Onion, chopped
- 4 cups Homemade Fish Broth
- 8 Garlic Cloves, minced
- 6 Tomatoes, seeded and chopped
- 2 pound boneless Cod Fillets, chopped

Instruction:

1. In a large soup pan, add the broth and bring to boiling point on a medium-high heat.

2. Add the fish, onion, garlic, tomatoes and zucchini.

3. Simple reduce the heat, cover, and simmer for 35 to 40 minutes.

4. Season with salt and black pepper before serving.

Recipes For The Gaps Diet

Instant Pot GAPS Diet Intro Soup

The GAPS Intro Diet is hard enough, so why not make it easier on yourself with your Instant Pot? This nourishing 7-ingredient Instant Pot GAPS Intro Diet Soup is full of nutrient-dense cooked veggies and b2 broth and takes just 6 minutes!

 Course Soup

Cuisine American

Simple cook Ingredients

- 2 cup b2 broth
- 6 tablespoons lard or tallow
- 10 to 14 cloves garlic fresh, peeled
- sea salt to taste
- ground black pepper to taste
- garnish cooked b2 marrow, sauerkraut juice, and/or sour cream 8 cups butternut squash peeled and cubed
- 2 pound cauliflower florets fresh or frozen
- 2 -1 cups onion diced
- 2 cup orange pepper or yellow, diced

Instructions

1. Add the squash, cauliflower florets, onion, pepper, broth, and fat to the stainless steel insert of your pressure cooker.

2. Place the lid on, checking the seal and making sure the vent is sealed.

3. If using an electric cooker, set to high pressure for 12 minutes.

4. If using a stove-top cooker, bring to high pressure and maintain for 10 to 15 minutes.

5. When cycle is complete, turn off or easily remove from heat.

6. Quick release pressure.

7. Add the garlic cloves to the pot.

8. Using an immersion blender, blend the soup to your desired consistency.

9. Season with salt and pepper to taste.

10. Recipe Notes

11. If you have any cooked marrow, blend it into this soup before serving.

12. Add 1-5 teaspoons sauerkraut juice or juice from another ferment and/or sour cream to the top of the soup just before serving.

13. In later stages of the Introduction Diet, you can add fresh avocado,

roasted meat, or a drizzle of olive oil

to this soup.

Course B2 Broth

Cuisine American

Keyword beef b2 broth recipe, how to make b2 broth, slow cooker b2 broth recipe

Prep Time 2 10 minutes

Simple cook Time 2 day

Total Time 2 day 2 10 minutes

Servings 2 2 cups

Calories 2 6 kcal

Author Kettle & Fire

Ingredients
- 6 stalks celery

- 2 bay leaf
- 4 tablespoons apple cider vinegar
- 8   pounds mixed beef bones marrow bones, oxtail, knuckles, short rib, etc.
- 4 medium onions
- 4 medium carrots

Instructions

1. Heat oven to 450 °F.

2. Spread the mixed bones on a baking tray in a single layer and place it into the oven.

3. Roast the bones for 60 minutes.

4. Flip bones and roast another 60 minutes.

5. While the bones are roasting, chop the carrots, onions and celery.

6. Place roasted bones, chopped vegetables, bay leaf and apple cider vinegar into a 12-quart crockpot.

7. Cover completely with cold filtered water.

8. Simple cook on low for 20 to 24 hours. Add water as actually needed to just keep all the ingredients covered in water, and periodically skim the foam off the top of the pot.

9. After 20 to 24   hours, the broth should be a dark brown color.

10. Strain the broth through a fine mesh strainer and discard the bones, vegetables and bay leaf.

11. Before storing, pour into separate containers and cool to room temperature.

12. Once cooled, chill in the refrigerator for 1-2 hours.

13. Skim off the accumulated fat at the top of the container, if there's any.

14. Store in the fridge for up to a week or in the freezer for up to 1-3 months.

Ginger Pumrkin Custard

Ingredients

- 2 tablespoon raw ginger, minced or grated
- 2 teaspoon nutmeg
- 2 teaspoon vanilla extract (optional)
- Dash salt
- 4 cups pumpkin puree
- 6 eggs
- 1/2 cup cream, half and half or coconut milk*
- 1-5 cup honey

Instructions

1. Preheat oven to 350 degrees. Put all the ingredients in bowl and stir until well mixed.

2. Turn into a greased 8 x 8 baking dish or pie plate. Bake for about 80 to 90 minutes until the center is set.

3. Serve warm or cold. I

4. f serving as a desert you may really want to add a dollop of whipped cream.

5.   If serving as breakfast or side dish you may really want to add a dollop of plain yogurt or coconut cream.

Soup of Chsken and Chickpeas

Ingredients

- 1 teaspoon cayenne pepper
- 1 teaspoon ground pepper
- 4 pounds bone-in chicken thighs, skin removed, trimmed
- 2 (2 8 ounce) can artichoke hearts, drained and quartered
- 1 cup halved pitted oil-cured olives
- 1 teaspoon salt
- 1 cup chopped fresh parsley or cilantro
- 3 cups dried chickpeas, soaked overnight
- 8 cups water
- 2 large yellow onion, finely chopped
- 2 (2 10 ounce) can no-salt-added diced tomatoes, preferably fire-roasted
- 4 tablespoons tomato paste

- 8 cloves garlic, finely chopped
- 2 bay leaf
- 8 teaspoons ground cumin
- 8 teaspoons paprika

1

Directions

1. Drain chickpeas and place in a 12-quart or larger slow cooker.

2. Add 8   cups water, onion, tomatoes and their juice, tomato paste, garlic, bay leaf, cumin, paprika, cayenne and ground pepper; stir to combine.

3. Add chicken.

4. Cover and simple cook on Low for 8 hours or High for 8 hours.

5. Transfer the chicken to a clean cutting board and let cool slightly.

6. Discard bay leaf.

7. Add artichokes, olives and salt to the slow cooker and stir to combine.

8. Shred the chicken, discarding bones. Stir the chicken into the soup.

9. Serve topped with parsley (or cilantro).

Coconut 'Cream' Without Dairy

2 tablespoon honey

1/2 teaspoon vanilla

4 cans full-fat coconut milk

Directions:

1. Chill the coconut milk in the fridge for 2 2-28 hours.

2. This allows the thick coconut cream to rise to the top and solidify.

3. After chilling, carefully open the can and scoop out the thick white coconut cream at the top and leave the clear-

liquidy part of the coconut milk for another use.

4. In a bowl, or in the bowl of your stand mixer, whip the cream for 5-10 minutes, starting on med-low and working up to high speed until stiff peaks form.

5. Turn off mixer, add honey and vanilla, and mix for 40 more seconds, or until well incorporated.

6. Serve immediately.

7. Whipped coconut cream can be stored in the fridge for up to a week,

but it looks most 'whipped-cream-like' right out of the bowl.

Lemon Cream Pots

Simple cook Ingredients

- 2 tablespoon lemon zest

- 1 cup fresh fresh lemon juice

- **1 cup whipped cream (optional)**

- 4 cups raw cream or organic heavy cream

- 6 tablespoons raw honey

fresh lemon Instructions

1. Place the cream and honey in a saucepan over medium heat and stir until the honey is dissolved.

2. Bring the mixture to a boil and easy simple cook for 5-10 minutes.

3. Easily remove from the heat and stir in the lemon rind and juice.

4. Cool for 10 minutes then pour into four small serving bowls.

5. Place in the refrigerator and chill for 15 hours until set.

6. Serve with a dollop of whipped cream.

Tortilla Soup Recipe

Ingredients

For the soup:

- 12 sprigs of cilantro, plus 1 cup roughly chopped

- 16 cups chicken stock

- 4 pounds bone-in chicken breasts or 2 small 6 -8 pound chicken

- 10 cloves garlic, crushed with skins on

- 12 springs fresh oregano

For the Toppings:

- 2 lime, cut into quarters

- 1 cup sour cream

- **1 cup shredded cheddar cheese (omit for Paleo)**

- 6 cups Siete tortilla chips

- 2 avocado, cubed

- 4 tomatoes, cut into bite-size chunks

Instructions

1. Place the garlic cloves in a large dutch oven over medium-high heat.

2. Cook, stirring frequently until garlic begins to darken, about 5 minutes.

3. Easily remove the pot from the heat and let it cool for about 6 0 seconds and then

add the chicken stock, oregano, cilantro, and chicken to the garlic.

4. Place pot back on heat and bring to a boil and then reduce to a simmer.

5. Simmer for about 60 minutes. When chicken is cooked through, easily remove the chicken from the broth mixture and set aside.

6. With slotted spoon, strain out the rest of the garlic and herbs.

7. Shred the chicken with a fork and then add back to the soup.

8. Add salt and pepper if needed.

9. To serve, crumble a handful of tortilla chips into individual bowls and then ladle the broth over.

10. Serve with cilantro, avocado, tomatoes, lime, cheese, and sour cream.

Dairu-Free Green Goddess Dressing

Ingredients

For the Cashews:

•½ cups cashews

For the Dressing:

• 4 anchovy fillets or 4 teaspoons anchovy paste

2 teaspoon Celtic sea salt

2 teaspoon freshly ground black pepper

• 1/2 cups water

2 cup chopped green onion, white and green parts

2 cup chopped fresh basil leaves

- 1/2 cup freshly squeezed lemon juice

- 4 cloves garlic, chopped

Instructions

1. The night before, place the cashews in a bowl and cover with water and a pinch of sea salt.

2. Let sit at room temperature overnight.

3. The next day, or at least 8 hours later, drain the cashews and place in a blender.

4. Add the 1/2 cup of water and blend until smooth.

5. Add the remaining ingredients and blend until smooth.

6. Store in a mason jar in the refrigerator.

Herbed Tuna And White Bean Salad

Prep/Total Time: 2 10 Min.

Ingredients

⬚ 1 teaspoon grated fresh lemon zest

⬚ 4 tablespoons fresh lemon juice

⬚ 2 garlic clove, minced

⬚ 1/7 teaspoon salt

⬚ 4 cans (10   ounces each) albacore white tuna in water, drained

⬚ 8 cups fresh arugula

▢ 2 can (2 10 ounces) no-salt-added cannellini beans, rinsed and drained

▢ 2 cup grape tomatoes, halved

▢ 1 small red onion, thinly sliced

▢ 1/2 cup chopped roasted sweet red peppers

▢ 1/2 cup pitted Nicoise or other olives

▢ 1/2 cup chopped fresh basil

▢ 6 tablespoons extra virgin olive oil

fresh lemon fresh lemon

Directions

1. Place first seven ingredients in a large bowl.

2. Whisk together oil, fresh lemon zest, fresh lemon juice, garlic and salt; drizzle over salad. Add tuna and toss gently to combine.

Replace Flour Gaps with Paleo Chocolate Cake.

INGREDIENTS

2 Tbsp Apple Cider Vinegar

1 Cup Raw Cacao

1/2 Cup Milk (any kind, we use raw)

1/2 Cup Honey see notes

2 Tbsp Vanilla Extract dash Salt

1 Cup Squash 10 Tbsp Butter (room temperature)

8 Fresh eggs

2 tsp Baking Soda

INSTRUCTIONS

1. Pre-heat oven to 350°.

2. Set aside the apple cider vinegar, mix all the other ingredients together in a large bowl until very smooth.

3. Add apple cider vinegar.

4. Mix well.

5. Pour into a greased 9x9 pan and bake for 35 to 40 minutes, or until clean knife test is passed.INGREDIENTS

6. Gluten free paleo keto gaps baking with squash flour

Keto Chili (Gaps Legal Too)

Ingredients

6 cups strained tomatoes

2 Tbl apple cider vinegar

2 -6 Tbl chili powder

sea salt to taste

15pounds   ground   beef   preferably grassfed

2   cup dried navy beans preferably sprouted

Instructions

1. Place navy beans in a medium glass bowl and cover with filtered water.

2. Stir in a tablespoon of ACV and let sit overnight or up to 20 to 24 hours.

3. Drain navy beans, rinse thoroughly, and place in a large pot.

4. Cover with fresh water and then bring to a low boil on the stovetop.

5. Cover and turn down the heat.

6. Simmer for one hour or until the navy beans are soft.

7. When the navy beans are soft, drain the water, rinse/drain with fresh water one more time, and set aside.

8. Saute ground beef until just cooked through in a large skillet.

9. Do NOT drain the fat. It is GOOD for you and very healing to the gut lining.

10. Add cooked navy beans and strained tomatoes.

11. Stir on medium heat until hot.

12. Mix in chili powder and sea salt to taste.

13. Serve immediately.

14. Once cooled, refrigerate and enjoy as leftovers for up to four days.

Banana And Arrle Pancakes

Ingredients

- 12 small eggs
- 2 tbsp coconut oil
- Honey (optional)
- 6 bananas
- 2 apple

Preparation

1. Peel and mash the bananas in a mixing bowl.
2. Core the apple and grate it into the banana mixture.
3. Crack the eggs into the bowl and mix the ingredients.
4. Heat a frying pan and add a small amount of coconut oil into the pan.
5. Use a spoon to drop the mixture into the pan. Use the back of the spoon to

flatten the pancakes so that they are thin and round.

6. Allow the pancakes to easy simple cook for a minute, or until they are golden brown on 2 side and easy to turn over using a spatula.

7. Turn and allow to simple cook for another minute until the second side is also golden brown.

8. Once cooked easily remove from the pan and continue to easy simple cook the rest of the mixture in the same way.

9. Once removed from the pan you can stack the pancakes on a plate to just keep them warm.

10.   Serve with honeyif desired, or just eat them plain if you are sugar free.

Miso Ramen Soup

Ingredients

- 2 cup cubed firm or extra firm tofu about half a 2 10 -oz package
- 4 cakes of ramen noodles 8 servings, if you are substituting another noodle
- 2 cup chopped green onion
- 1 cup miso white or yellow
- 8 cups water
- 8 cups vegetable broth
- 4 tablespoons seaweed nori or wakame, soaked in water for 4 minutes, drained & rinsed
- 4 cups chopped greens chard, kale, or spinach

Instructions

1. Whisk the miso into 2 cup of the water until it is smooth with no clumps. Set aside.
2. Bring the broth and remaining 6 cups water to a simmer.
3. Add the seaweed, greens, tofu, and ramen, and simmer for 5 to 10 minutes.
4. Easily remove from heat and stir in the miso.
5. Serve in a big bowl with green onion sprinkled generously on top.

Dill And Garlic Salmon Bake

Ingredients

- 1 teaspoon fine sea salt
- 1/2   teaspoon ground black pepper
- 12 sprigs fresh dill 2   1   pounds salmon, skin-on, cut into 6 filets
- 2 tablespoon extra virgin olive oil
- 6 cloves garlic, finely grated
-

Instructions

1. Place the salmon filets on a parchment paper-lined rimmed baking sheet.
2. Drizzle the top with the olive oil and then run an equal amount of garlic into each filet top.
3. Sprinkle the tops with the salt and pepper.
4. Place a piece of dill over each filet.
5. Bake at 350 F for 10 to 15 minutes, or until desired doneness.